I0425534

# THIS NOTEBOOK BELONGS TO:

______________________________

www.ingramcontent.com/pod-product-compliance
Lightning Source LLC
Chambersburg PA
CBHW051356280526
45784CB00007B/2978
* 9 7 8 1 0 9 0 4 9 3 2 4 8 *